25 TIPS

for

SURVIVING ALZHEIMER'S

Lisa Cerasoli

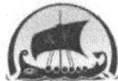

STORY MERCHANT BOOKS
LOS ANGELES • 2019

25 Tips for Surviving Alzheimer's

ISBN-13: 978-0-9963689-9-5

Story Merchant Books
400 S. Burnside Avenue, #11B
Los Angeles, CA 90036
www.storymerchantbooks.com

www.529Books.com
Interior Design: Lauren Michelle
Cover: Claire Moore

25 TIPS

for
SURVIVING ALZHEIMER'S

...and More Confessions from a Caregiver

Lisa Cerasoli

Mission Statement

I survived caring for someone with Alzheimer's.

I could tell you that it's easy, but it's not.

I could say you'll get lots of medals and pats on the back for a job well done, but you won't.

Family will surround you and shower you with love, support, and humor. They'll chip in! I could say that, but it's not always the case.

And I could add that afterwards you can check being awesome off your bucket list…and call it good. But you won't do that: Once a caregiver always a caregiver. Once you discover it, you can't *undiscover* that quality inside you—the ability to give care to someone in need. And you'll probably do it again….

What I can tell you is this: chances are you won't be showered with accolades because of your sacrifices. In fact, the opposite could happen. People might hate you for it. (Yes, I just used the "h" word.) *She's in it for the money. He's lazy.* That's what they could say. Because why you're really doing it—the real reason—can be impossible for some to understand.

Love, compassion, sacrifice: those are just words to some people, just like they used to be words to me, until I had to put them into use. I lost friends because of love, compassion, and sacrifice. I lost family members. It made me sad and so I cried. Sometimes I still do. But I'd do it all over again to help someone I love.

When I look back at the last seven years of my grandmother's life, I know she was safe, and that's important. But above and beyond that, I know she was loved. My daughter did that, my former husband did that, my stepson did that, and I did my best to do that— to love somebody who needed someone to hang on, so she could safely let go. We hung on.

We're different now. We have a secret, a bond; we know what the other is capable of. We don't all live together anymore. But we have an unbreakable respect for each other. We don't talk about it much, our caregiving days, but it's in our eyes and our actions. It's ingrained. Even if we are simply saying hello in passing, the energy of that experience surfaces. Our compassion connects us; that's because of Nora Jo.

We survived Alzheimer's.

I wish I could say that my marriage survived Alzheimer's.

And I want to tell everyone that once you're neck high in caregiving you'll get the swing of it and get good at it. You'll be able to care for someone with a dementia-related illness like it's second nature, like driving. But it's not like that. Alzheimer's is unpredictable; it's the opposite of stopping when the light turns red and going when it's green. I never perfected the business of caregiving. The thing that kept me going was a personal need to finish every race I've ever started, and a deep maternal love as Gram grew to need me more by thy day. Don't expect others to do what you do. Everybody's best is different. Don't expect everyone to understand. Do get help when it's available. This is not a one-person job. There's no room for ego in caregiving.

I survived Alzheimer's.

Even though my marriage didn't make it, my former partner, Jazzy's dad, survived it, too. I never could have pulled that off alone. Nora Jo wasn't his grandmother. That didn't change over time. But, they did become best friends. He's a survivor. Big time.

My daughter is a survivor.

My stepson is a survivor.

...And you can be, too.

This is a story about surviving Alzheimer's.
We have survived it...so far.
But until we find a cure, only time will tell.

Dedication

This book is dedicated to all caregivers.

In my memoir, *As Nora Jo Fades Away*, I wrote: "Between my young, daughter, Jazz, my Tea Cup Poodle, Beau, and my gram, Miss Nora Jo, I haven't peed alone since the summer of '05."

It's been nearly a decade since Gram passed, and I miss her every day. I miss my "entourage." I miss having something to always do. I get lonely for her still (although, not so much when I'm peeing). I understand the relief that comes when a caregiving job ends, and I'm aware of the dull ache that succeeds it. My grandmother is at peace. I know that. But that ache is a part of me now; it comes with my own sense of peace, and so I welcome it. I wouldn't have it any other way.

• • •

I want everyone to know that while you're busy caring, there are tons of us out here in this big, beautiful world rooting for you. Caregiving gets lonely. But there are new friends, neighbors you never really knew, and family members you weren't that close to that can help. Let's call them comrades in compassion. They're on the journey, too, but you have to stop and notice them. Start with a "hello." Like, the Alzheimer's Association and me—we're here to help, but you have to give us a shout.

I wrote *As Nora Jo Fades Away* while I was caregiving fulltime. *25 TIPS...* and the ensuing stories were compiled upon examination of that journey. While the two books share a similar message, I was in very different states of mind when I wrote them, which is reflected in their varying narrative tones. The purpose of this book is to bestow invaluable tips on the overworked, under slept caregiver—because back when I was in the thick of it and my family and I were fumbling blindly in our caregiving endeavors, we could have used a guide like this. And, so....

As an added bonus, there are 5 TIPS from my daughter, Jazz! Honestly, hers are the best—a child's perspective.

This book is for you.
Thank you so much for doing what you do.

—Lisa Cerasoli

Table of Contents

25 TIPS
for
SURVIVING ALZHEIMER'S

Backstory…for those who haven't read *Nora Jo.*

In the year 2000, I lived in Los Angeles as a working actor. I had three main concerns back then:

1. When was I going to book my next gig?
2. Where was I going to get my next sushi fix?
3. And, how many hours did I need to spend at the gym to compete this week?

That was then.

Then came the fall of 2002 when my father was diagnosed with stage four lung cancer. I left for Michigan and life got real—real scary. Cold, day-old pizza readily replaced sushi from my favorite five-star restaurant. A for the figure I worked so hard to maintain: it was hidden beneath a pair of sweats for the majority of 2003. My acting career vanished in a flash. I replaced *The Seven Habits of Highly* Effective *People* with *Conversations with God* and read that until the book became a mass of pink highlights. Then I read it aloud to Dad to quiet his mind—rereading the pink parts for emphasis. We became best friends in 2003. We were barely acquaintances before that.

I will never forget the day he said "you're so nice" with tears in his eyes.

I was massaging his feet because the cancer had gone into his bones—his spine and hip—and he was often in severe pain. I had discovered that even more than oxytocin and morphine, a foot massage could temporarily ease pain.

He told me I was nice, which was nice, and so I smiled. And then he said it for the second time: "You're so nice." And, as tears trailed from his eyes to his chin, he added, "I never knew that about you."

He died about a month later.

I was thirty-three. My dad never knew I was nice. If caregiving isn't the best anecdote for vanity, I don't know what is.

The next time you feel inferior because you need your hair done or your roots touched up or an hour at the gym or an afternoon at the lake with only your fishing pole, remember that you've turned in your *me first* card for an invisible halo. Okay, that's extreme. We're all just human. We're all doing our best here; I get that. But caregivers pull from a deep well of compassion in order to get through the days, months, years….

The amygdala (a network of nerves in the brain) has been shown to be larger in scans of altruistic people than it is in others.

Don't take what you do lightly. Don't confuse exhaustion with inferiority because life doesn't feel so perfect anymore.

People told me I was nice all the time when I lived in LA. I think that was because I was from the Midwest. I know I wasn't handing out foot massages back then that's for sure; it must've been because I was a Midwest girl. That's not why my dad said it, though.

We barely spoke before his diagnosis, my dad and me. We weren't mad at each other; there just never seemed to be anything to talk about. If I were to guess, I'd say my dad was surprised by my ability to care for him—this guy who was a stranger, mostly. I was, too.

The truth is when my father became ill, I went home for my mom. She's always been like a best friend to me. So, I went home to help her with Dad. I did not go home for him. Not for him. But, when I got there, it didn't take long to realize that this wasn't about a daughter helping her mother, or a daughter's last attempt to guilt Dad into getting to know her. This was about giving care and companionship to someone who was scared, alone, and in pain. This was about holding someone's hand while they faced death. The fact that he was my dad was secondary. That's what I realized when I got there. My job was to hold this person's hand, all day and night if necessary, and that was my only job. What happened, consequently, was we became best friends. For ten months, I had a new best friend.

That was cool.

And this new best friend reminded me about the things I had been forgetting in life: That how I looked didn't matter. That where I worked wasn't important: That my figure…was fine…or whatever. And that coffee tastes pretty good with or without cream—the cream was no longer the important part. My father, my friend, the guy whose hand I was holding and feet I was massaging, reacquainted me with what mattered.

And he reminded me that I was nice.

Looking back, I needed the good kick in the ass that caregiving gave me. I mean, there was more work for me on the horizon, obviously (Nora Jo). And, this, this time with my dad was what *they* call scratching the surface. My journey to becoming a more caring, compassionate person began with Dad....

By 2003, I was married. A year later I was pregnant. It happened fast! Jazzlyn Jo Weaver arrived on her due date: June 1, 2005. She had dark gorgeous wavy hair and her daddy's eyes. And it wasn't long before we realized she inherited her great grandmother's sense of humor. She was just as I had imagined in my dreams. And, life got busy, baby busy. Then, in 2006, my ever-so-witty grandmother, Miss Nora Jo, was officially diagnosed with Alzheimer disease. We moved her in until her death on December 16, 2010.

I fled to LA as a kid in search of my dreams but found them as a grown up in the very place from which I'd ran. I am consumed with love for my daughter and find total peace in caregiving, writing, and speaking about Alzheimer's. Deepak Chopra says that this is taking *karma* and turning it into *dharma*. Dharma is when passion finds purpose. I've taken an adverse situation and discovered it was, in fact, my purpose in life. For that I think I'm lucky, crazy lucky. I thank God for these offbeat circumstances—for my life—every day.

Sometimes the exhaustion and redundancy of caregiving can muddy up the vision we have for ourselves and our futures. I know that feeling well. If you're feeling cloudy, this is a quick reminder that life, however difficult, has purpose. You're saving someone every time you rise to care for them. I'm so thankful to be so capable. I'm grateful for you—that there's so many of you who care. And even if they can't express it—the people you're caring for—they're grateful too. I know that for fact. When there was nothing else there, I still saw that in my grandmother's eyes.

First cancer but ultimately Alzheimer's disease and caregiving in general has opened my eyes and heart to a world that was foreign. Despite nearly a decade worth of experience under my belt, I'm still a pup, a newborn looking on in fascination and sadness at the oddities of dementia-related illnesses. I can't count all the days where the challenges of caregiving booted me behind a closed door where I cursed and cried. But truth be told, I've always been a bit of a potty mouth and a drama queen, so that might just be me. The thing is I made it; I'm still in one piece.

And, I work out regularly: yoga, weights, running, floor hockey, hiking. But, I've made that an important part of my routine to help me shape my mind and heart as much as my body—to teach me how to be still so I can think, breathe, care, and laugh through the struggles of caregiving, disease, and the inevitable: death.

Thanks to caregiving, I've learned not to plan ahead too much. But I always plan to be inspired, entertained, and educated—those are the kinds of plan I make in life now.

Thanks to my gram, I now communicate through books, blogs, film, and speaking engagements to the growing community of caregivers in this world. I have finally "let go" and found freedom in compassion. Compassion is cool. Plus, in doing this, I'm honoring a woman who was my idol. She will always be my hero. All I did by caring for her was pay it back.

5 TIPS to Get Organized

1. CLUTTER CLEAR. Get rid of breakables and valuables like vases, ornaments, glassware. Remove loose rugs, or tape them securely down. Move pictures that could be knocked off a shelf, toys from the ground (have a bin in a corner if necessary) and move shoes that are usually left out randomly (bin). Give everything "a home," just like you're giving your loved one a home.

2. FAMILIARIZE their surroundings with as much memorabilia from their old life as possible. Move in their own bed, dressers, books, lamps, etc., if possible. Have a TV in the bedroom (if they enjoy that). Label *on*, *off*, *volume* on remote, if they can still use it.

3. Create AMPLE SPACE in the BATHROOM for their toiletries. It is crucial they have their own space, and know their personal belongings are with them, too.

4. Create a SPOT in the MAIN LIVING AREA for the person you're caring for. It may be a tray

(or table) next to a comfortable chair (or rocker) with a Kleenex box, a magazine or book, along with their favorite mug.

5. Teach the person you're caring for where everything is in your kitchen. People are used to maneuvering easily in a kitchen. Even knowing they'll forget, put the essentials on the counter (like coffee), so they don't feel completely lost yet. Demonstrate repeatedly how simple it is to find food and drink items in your kitchen. Eyelevel is key here. If you place the coffee on the counter, they'll feel good about finding it. Anything they can do on their own puts them at ease.

The Bread Story

Over the last three years of full-time caregiving, we had turned into The House of Notes. I don't just mean of the milk-eggs-bread sort. If any of you have watched my Survival Tips Videos with Leeza Gibbons, or seen my film, you know that notes have graced many a wall at the Weaver-Cerasoli joint:

○ *Bathroom This Way.*
○ *Gram, This is Your Bedroom.*
○ *Gram, your little boy is not lost. He is safe with me. Love, Lisa*
○ *Please Don't Feed the Dogs, They will Die. Thanks!*
○ *No Beer Cans in the Microwave. Thanks!*
○ *Gram, if the Shower is on, Please Don't Open the Curtain and say, "Hi." Thanks!*

Those were just a few.

I also had some others that resided in a kitchen drawer:

○ *I'll be Home Soon. Love, Lisa*
○ *Went to Gym, be Back in 5 Minutes. And…*
○ *Went to Buy Bread, be Back in 5 Minutes. Love, Lisa*

Somehow, that last one—The Bread Note—kept ending up at the top of the pile. And because of Gram's Alzheimer disease, I assumed it didn't matter which note I used, as long as (if she got up and read it) she'd know I'd be home soon. So, the I'm-out-buying-bread note became the standard for about three weeks. I thought nothing of it.

Spring 2010

I slipped into my yoga pants, grabbed a boiled egg from the fridge, filled a plastic bottle with water, opened the note drawer, took out the I'm-out-buying-bread note, and placed it next to the coffee pot:

Gram, Went to Buy Bread, be Back in 5 Minutes.
Love, Lisa

And then I high-tailed it to the gym.

One Hour Later

I met our part-time caregiver at the door and entered just behind her.

Gram was at the counter pouring a cup of coffee. I was still in the entryway taking off my boots and jacket when I heard her say, "Oh, hi, honey," to the part-time caregiver. Then she said, "Lisa's out buying bread. Again. I swear, all that girl does these days is buy bread. You'd think it might occur to her to grab two goddamned loaves the next time she goes to the store!" Then she let out a big laugh and tagged that with; "Maybe one of us ought to tell her!" After one final bellow shot out her mouth, she uttered, "…Or not!" and nearly doubled over giggling.

I walked in (blushing). There was my gram, holding up the bread note for all to see.

And there was me—looking like a breadless fool.

A woman with moderate-to-advanced Alzheimer's disease—a woman I gave way too little credit to—was onto me. It was downright embarrassing, and well worth a belly laugh or two.

As they say in the movie, *Dan in Real Life*: "Plan to be surprised."

I was surprised.

All I thought as I stood there embarrassed by my eighty-nine-year-old grandmother is, you're never too old to learn…and apparently never too young, either! I learned quite a lesson that morning.

These notes, however funny, did manage to keep my gram safe, and relieved a lot of her anxiety. They were true lifesavers. The don't feed the dogs sign saved the life of our Tea Cup Poodle, Beau! (You're welcome, Beau.) It really did; he was three pounds and couldn't handle people food.

If I can become a caregiver, you can too.

My grandmother, Nora Jo, moved in with my family in 2007 when her Alzheimer's disease advanced to the point where it was dangerous for her to live alone. That's when "chaos" of ultra-farcical proportions began, or, "Life went from Michigan to Mars," as I've been known to say. But the illness brought moments of joy, too. As odd as that sounds, we all became closer, we learned to survive, we learned the true meaning of love, and discovered laughter in the craziest of places: sometimes on a post-it taped to the microwave.

5 SAFETY TIPS for Caregiving

1. You know it: SIGNS. Most people can READ well into Alzheimer's. Don't be shy—label everything. We even put three colorful signs trailing each other down the hallway to the bathroom with big arrows underneath the words. Gram didn't have an accident for a long time after that. These signs make great conversation pieces too. And don't forget, you can always put a picture on a sign.

2. Buy cheap BABY GATES to protect against stairs and doorways.

3. Buy childproof SAFTEY LOCKS for doors. My five-year-old, Jazz, had these figured out in two seconds, but Gram never did.

4. Place unsafe items in HIGH PLACES. Very low places can work too. These spots are outside of the line of vision, which means they're outside of the reality of a person with Alzheimer's.

5. USER-FRIENDLY ITEMS should be at EYELEVEL and within arm's reach: towels,

tissues, snacks. Limit the amount, though. You don't want eight Kleenex boxes opened at once, or two-dozen Nutter Butters gone from the pack before anyone else gets a shot at them. (Sorry, Jazz!)

*Eat, Pray, Love...*and my Grandma's Bra

In the fall of 2010, after six years of part- and full-time caregiving, I noticed my Grandma's bras were starting to drive her nuts. There were a number of logical reasons for this. The biggest reason was they were from a different era (literally). Yet, they had magically managed to travel through time, and somehow maintain enough composure to survive seven decades, but not quite enough to still be functional. I didn't know what size they were as the tags were all faded and frayed. And the band around every bra was so stretched that when unlatched, they appeared completely rippled. The darted effect—so reminiscent of her time—had stayed intact, but that was about it.

Needless to say, she needed new bras in what I guesstimated to be a size 40A (for all you dudes out there who are unfamiliar with this measurement, it's primarily because it doesn't exist). Because of Alzheimer's disease, she needed new bras

that worked just like the old ones. She had no understanding of what to do with sports bras that went over the head, and the thought of not wearing one was sacrilege.

Ah, a new mission had arisen.

About every two months, I was faced with an interesting and eccentric new task as caregiver. Buying Gram a slew of new bras had become The Mission of The Fall of 2010, and Jazz was thrilled.

This project took weeks. In that time, Jazz and I brought home no fewer than eighteen bras—sizes 36A, 38B, 38C. They were too big, too small, and no amount of convincing could assure Gram to settle for any one of them.

At one point, Jazz said, "G.G., why don't you put them in your drawer in your drawer for next year. That's what I do when Mama buys me clothes that don't fit; I wait a year and grow into them!"

Her point was brilliant, so I ran with it, too. But Gram wasn't buying the B.S. we were selling. We ultimately gave up.

It was a Saturday night around Halloween. Jazz had a party, my husband was gone to a friend's cottage (hunting season), and I wanted to see a movie. *Eat, Pray, Love* was playing. I figured, even if Gram didn't understand the movie, she could enjoy nice music and beautiful cinematography for a couple of hours. It was a Julia Roberts flick; they're generally appealing to the senses and harmless in every other way. A friend joined us. We were the last to walk into the theater with Gram in tow. We brought along a big, wool blanket, and then tucked her into her theatre seat nice 'n cozy, like good caregivers do. We could hear people "ooh" and "aah" and comment on how cute we all were.

And then....

Well, Gram possessed neither an inside voice, nor a new bra yet—two things I hadn't factored into our movie going experience.

So, about ten minutes into the movie, Gram shouted (and I do mean shouted), "Honey, unhook my bra! It's cutting the shit out of me!"

So that happened.

A quiet theatre had suddenly been roused. A serene movie had turned instantaneously slapstick. I almost peed but crossed my legs efficiently and dove inside the back of her series of sweaters and thermals to remedy the situation.

She kept repeating herself over, and over, too. It was really bothering her (plus...the Alzheimer's).

I worked like a madwoman to stifle my boisterous gram who

had started uttering, "Lower! The goddamned hook is lower!"

I finally found "the g*$#@*^#d hook." It was tucked and stuck inside the back of the waistband of her underpants. I couldn't help but sympathize with the woman. I mean, if the back of my bra was hooked onto my undies, I'd be uncomfortable too.

I then peeled my friend off the floor. She was laughing that hard. And we all resumed our movie watching.

Overall, I believe the incident enhanced everyone's *Eat, Pray, Love* experience. And the line should be written into the show. It did, after all, get the biggest laugh.

That night I went home and indulged in a little drink, pray, love.

The next day I left the house on a mission: to find at least two bras in the size 40A. Thank you, Kohl's— mission accomplished. Oh, and thank you, God. There's never a dull moment in the land of Nora Jo.

If you're ever feeling like your moments as a caregiver are dull, stifling, and uneventful, I hope you think of this story, and maybe come up with one of your own. I believe, above all, humor is a powerful tool. We could've been embarrassed by my gram's antics in the theater, but we chose to laugh instead. The result? People laughed along with us.

5 More Safety TIPS

1. SEGREGATE YOUR PETS (if you have any) from the person you're caring for IF these pets are a "road hazard." Pets under the feet are the number one cause of accidents in the home—the number one cause. They are especially dangerous for people who can't remember they exist. Doing this at night is extra important, as it's harder to spot them. A baby gate works great for this purpose. Put it between the kitchen and living room, for example, and keep your pets restricted to a smaller part of the house, like the kitchen at night.

2. NIGHTLIGHTS. Buy a ton of nightlights. Invest in the stock if it'll make you feel better! Use them all over; in rooms they may wander into, near your signs, to light all hallways. We had fourteen nightlights. It was just enough in our three-bedroom home to help everyone sleep a bit more soundly.

3. Use PLASTIC glassware. Your loved one is klutzy. Heck, I'm klutzy. Go plastic. That was difficult for me, as I prefer glass, but it saved me

from cleaning up a lot of messes…and it reduced stress.

4. HIDE ALCOHOL and…
5. PRESCRIPTION DRUGS. I lost a week's worth of penicillin because it was left on the counter as a morning reminder.

40/40 Vision

Name one thing that's hard to do when you're in your forties. I'm not talking about the splits or getting carded—but I have noticed that doing the splits is becoming increasingly difficult (even with all my yoga) and getting carded seems to be a thing of the past (insert sad face). I'm talking about making new friends. That would be #1 on my list for things that become harder to do as life goes on. It's hard to make new friends while your life is consumed with jobs, kids, bills, spouses, school functions, trips, laundry—it's hard. When I make a new friend nowadays, I'm shocked. The first thing I think is, will this stick? Do either of us have time to devote to a new friendship? The answer usually turns out to be no. If making new and lasting friendships in your forties is rare like getting carded, can you imagine making new friends in your eighties? Can you imagine doing it while you're dying from Alzheimer's?

I keynoted about a dozen caregiver conferences in 2013. Jazz, who was eight at the time, along with my mother, Sheri, came to the last one of the year. I thought they were going to drop me off, but they walked in to pee, and decided to stay for the festivities. In truth, I think they saw the amazing spread and couldn't help themselves. Anyway, with Jazz in the room, ready-made speech flipped on its head.

The plan was to headline for an hour and then show our 29-minute documentary, *14 DAYS with Alzheimer's*. Well, I couldn't have been at the podium with mic in hand for more than a few minutes when Jazz raised her hand.

Naturally, I called on her.

"Um, yes, Jazz? Do…you have a question?"

"Yeah! Mom, you have to tell everyone the story about G.G. stealing the red cup from Applebee's! That story's awesome!"

I held back a laugh. "Okay, Jazz, I'll tell that story."

And so, I did.

And everyone enjoyed it.

I looked down at my notes, still on track.

I continued.

Five Minutes Later

Jazzy's hand flew up.

"Um, yes, Jazz?"

"You need to tell everyone about the time we tried to fit G.G. into my jogger stroller so we could walk to the park!"

And, I digressed to incorporate the stroller story—a tale that was equally as amusing.

Five Minutes Later

"Um, yes, Jazz?"

"Mom, I got your favorite dessert from the buffet table: Lemon bars! Grandma Sheri said they're your fave. Do you want one now?"

"Um, no, Jazz. I'm speaking, sweetheart. And, listen, you need to let Momma get through this; these folks have taken time out from their busy day to be here. If you keep raising your hand, we're all going to put you into a collective time-out? Got it?"

Everyone laughed.

(That was my best joke of the night.)

My keynote speech had turned interactive. I felt like I was back in college doing dinner theatre. The only thing missing was the wine. I had another five minutes before the movie was to start. I had a plan about to how to wrap up; I always had a plan…*but you know what they say*….

Jazz raised her hand.

I called on her.

"Mom, tell everyone how much fun her funeral was!"

I have a stockpile of stories from my adventures in caregiving. I could fill Packer Stadium with them. This wasn't one of them. Jazz was the first person to ever put the "fun" in funeral. This clearly meant something to her. I took the comment seriously, as Jazz lived through this too; life with Gram and Alzheimer's. She had what people refer to as an accelerated emotional maturity from being born into caregiving. She was one of the most in tune people I knew, and she said G.G.'s funeral was fun….

I thought about it, and about the word fun. I thought for a minute about all the people who showed up unexpectedly. I thought about the love, the conversations, the hugs, the tears, and the funny stories that were shared. The toasts that were made after the wake at a local pub, all in her honor, I remembered those. I remembered the classic country music blaring from the jukebox—Johnny Cash and Dolly Parton. Cans of warm Busch Light (G.G.'s favorite beer) were drank by all. People danced, laughed, cried, thanked me for the opportunity to know her. The room was bustling with joy from these comrades in compassion.

And that's when I developed this perfect *40/40 Vision* about Nora Jo's funeral and understood my daughter's comment.

My gram's death was somewhat unexpected. She spent a week dying in my home, but prior to her heart attack, Alzheimer's aside, she was fine. It's intense to have someone dying in a bed in your entryway—unable to speak or move. Many of you know this.

I was tired. I was emotionally and physically about as exhausted as I had ever been. I remembered her death; it happened at 9:10 a.m. on a Tuesday, just after Jazz kissed her goodbye and left for school. I remembered touching up her fingernails and toenails with her favorite pink polish, so she'd look pretty for her Fritz when she got to Heaven. I held up that guy—the one who carts off the dead people—so I could do that. I remembered putting together a quick hodgepodge video—an *In Memory Of*— to Dolly Parton's "I Will Always Love You" on the way to the wake (which was eighty miles out of town). I remembered thinking, man, I hope I'm going to Heaven and not that other place after this fiasco—the caregiving fiasco that took place in my home, in front of my young daughter and step kid, Brock.

There I was, sitting by her coffin, gazing down at her beauty and the peacefulness that magically exuded from her spiritless body.

That's when Jazz grabbed my arm. "Mom, look!"

Oh, look at that—some of our friends from out-of-town walked in.

"I'm going to go say, 'hi'!" she said, and off she dashed.

I waved. Before I lowered my hand, some more friends walked in; they were trailed by the Alzheimer's Association. Wow. They drove eighty miles to say goodbye too. Wow.

I looked around the room and decided to start counting. There must have been forty of our friends there, and they were all about forty years old. And my gram hadn't known a single one of them before she was diagnosed with Alzheimer's.

I was one of those forty-year-olds. In the last ten years of my life, I hadn't made forty new friends, not real ones that would travel like this to see me, not that I knew of, anyway. It's hard to make new friends as an adult.

My gram never had a driver's license. She barely left the house, even when she was strong and healthy. My gram spent the last six years of her life dying from a broken heart over the loss of my grandfather, Fritz, and from Alzheimer's disease. And my gram, somehow, made forty new friends that were half her age during that time too.

I was in awe. I was reminded of the power of God. If she were here, she wouldn't know any of these people.

But they knew her.

I know what you're thinking; they came for me, and for the whole family. No, they didn't. They came for her. I know this because I'm not close with most of them now.

They came for her.

At a time when friends are typically few, if they're even alive at all, my gram attracted a pack of devoted followers who cared about her, supported her, listened to her, and most of all, loved her unconditionally. Jazz recognized that.

And those people made G.G.'s funeral fun.

I'm still clueless about how to find friends that stick, but my family and I sure did serve as the facilitators for my gram. At least there was that. At least we did that much. Maybe our caregiving fiasco wasn't a fiasco at all. Maybe it was exactly as it was supposed to be: crazy beautiful. We did the best we could. Maybe, just maybe, we did good.

You should have seen this wake; it was standing room only. And, damn, was it fun.

Five TIPS for Surviving Caregiving

1. LAUGH. Let's face it; some of this stuff is plain funny. Find your freedom and laugh about it. It's better than crying (again). "Laugh and the world laughs with you. Poop your pants and you stand alone." Jazz taught me that one.

2. Got a story? WRITE it down. Journaling expels anxiety, sadness, and frustration. It sets burdens temporarily free. It also preserves your personal story. It's amazing what one can forget during this stressful process. It's incredible to have a journal to fall back on for comfort, for a good laugh, a good cry, or to bring clarity. I can't say enough about this. If you can't stand journaling (if this sounds like homework), try taking pictures—keep a journal like that.

3. Find your ME TIME. That phrase drove me nuts until I became a caregiver, then my free time, my me time, became precious as platinum. This can be a nap, a walk, a quick drink with a friend, one-hour worth of your favorite TV show

in silence. Maybe it means a game of cards with your significant other. Go to a movie!

4. And speaking of your significant other, how about a regularly scheduled DATE NIGHT…. This was not our idea, but we were talked into it, and it saved our third year of caregiving. It made us better caregivers and spouses.

5. EXERCISE. Endorphins are like fairy dust. Caregiving is a heavy-duty job. Give yourself a regular dose of gym-time or fresh air so you can fly again.

The Dread Zone

January 15, 2012

Lisa,

Hi. I just finished the book you wrote about your grandmother. And I just wanted to say, I should have never complained or felt exhausted. I only went to my dad's for a few hours every day. He didn't even live with me. I feel so wimpy. Thank you for changing my perspective. I'm glad I did what I did, but I wish it could have been more.

That note was waiting for me when I logged onto Facebook. I had never even met this woman; we weren't even FB friends. So many things went through my head.

- I felt sad that she felt terrible and "wimpy" about doing a good thing.
- Everybody's circumstances are different, and I didn't have a lot of details surrounding hers. And....
- Everybody's best is different.

I was a newbie in the world of part-time caregiving when this woman reached out. It had been two years since Gram had passed, and I had been assisting Mrs. Bennett for just three months now.

Prior to taking that job, I had thought my caregiving endeavors were over—that I'd filled my quota for this life (or at least this decade), put in overtime, paid my dues, all that jazz. Well, a friend needed part-time help. It was three hours daily. I had a flexible schedule. God knows I had the skills. The job had some pay, so there was that, I guess. And I really liked Mrs. Bennett; there was that, too. The questions were: Did I have the stamina? The desire? Compassion left to give? Part of me missed doing something for someone. Part of me thought that part-time caregiving would fill that void and be a synch. It's only part-time, after all…. That's why I accepted the job.

Having said that, I'm here to announce that steady, part-time caregiving is not easier than full-time work in your home. I know this now for fact. Sure, as a part-time caregiver, one gets to go home every day. I left. I was freed. But, I also had to come back the next day. And I often dreaded the coming back part. (Yes, I said "dread.") Some days, I dreaded it.

When you live with the person you're caring for, you're in a groove. You don't boomerang back and forth from the situation. You adapt differently. You don't' have to build up tolerance to do that thing you dread every day. I guess one might deduct that if you're caregiving full-time, you live right in the dread zone—but the truth is, you don't. Full-time caregivers don't live in the dread zone because they wouldn't survive it. They choose another tactic—they adapt to a world that doesn't appear to have a beginning or end, just a really long middle. They adjust to living in that vast middle of nowhere, somewhere, high energy, low energy, no energy, emergency, insomnia, exhaustion, hysteria, visitors (sometimes lots), help (sometimes poor), food (maybe, maybe not), beer (definitely—at least in my middle there was). That becomes the definition of their days, their lives, their jobs. And they're okay with that. Caregiving becomes one big long day. But it's not the sort of thing that is "dreaded," like winter, or doing your taxes, or getting a colonoscopy. There's no emotional buildup in full-time caregiving to produce a feeling of dread.

As a part-time caregiver, I got to sleep through the night. That was the biggest relief of all, but my lows became lower. They felt lower because of the ecstasy I felt upon escaping my daily duties, which conversely created the dread that consumed me moments prior to every return.

It only lasted for a moment, but it came upon me every day. I'd sit in my car with the engine off and stare at the house, her charming house. And I'd dread walking into the "same day" again. And then I'd take a deep breath, get over myself, and jump into the journey.

I don't think that one category of caregiving deserves less "honors" than the other, or deserves more, for that matter. I believe caregiving and caregivers do a good thing every day, whether it's for two hours, ten, or twenty-four. As a full-time caregiver, I often found myself running on fumes. Part-time caregivers refuel. They take that moment where they sit in their cars, take a deep breath, and then promise themselves to spend the next few hours giving one hundred percent.

There are a lot of incredible human beings in the world who can't adapt to caregiving at all. It's a special skill. It takes compassion, an open mind, the ability to adapt and let go, endurance. It's a marathon. I commend anybody who's been mastering the art of compassion, patience, tolerance, swallowing tears, and biting their tongue by being a caregiver at all. Period.

Let's not compete for "most hours logged." Let's just try and make every moment feel like a personal win by doing the best we can. I think the key to effective caregiving rarely lies in the big picture. It's captured in the tiny moments.

Think of it this way? Your "two hours," your 100% could be the highlight of their day. What a gift.

FIVE More TIPS for Surviving Caregiving

1. FIND BACKUP. Caregiving is NOT a one-person gig. Find someone, or an organization that can be there for you when you need a quick, unexpected escape.

2. PRAY. I'm serious. My best friend brought her family to meet Gram one summer, and she said, "Wow, you talk about God a lot. I don't remember you doing that in college." In college I only had my own life to worry about. Yeah, I did talk about God a lot, now that I thought about it. I talked *to* Him pretty regularly too.

3. Hold onto at least on favorite HOBBY. Whether it's reading, fishing, painting, collecting rocks, watching movies, walking the dog, gardening, cooking…incorporate your favorite thing to do into your weekly routine. Prioritize it. Remember, this job generally doesn't span the length of *your* life, so you need to have a life to go back to when this job is over.

4. BE SOCIAL and be social with your loved one. Everybody can't always do this, but if you can, get out of the house and into the world. Even if your loved one has drawn on their eyebrows with a bright blue Sharpie, and you don't notice until you're pulling into the parking lot at Apple Bees, suck it up and go in anyway. Enjoy your dinner! Ignore the looks! This will make for a great story (with or without the journaling). And, your loved one will enjoy the extra attention they receive from all the onlookers.

5. VENT. Maybe your backup person is the same person you can vent to but, if not, find someone trusting, and vent away. If you feel as though you don't have anyone, call the Alzheimer's Association. They have a 24-hour hotline: 1-800-272-3900. They're available seven days a week. They are incredible. They have saved my life on more than one occasion at 2:00 a.m. when I felt alone, frustrated, and lost.

Judge Judy and Mrs. B.

Aging has to be harder than any of us know, even us caregivers. Most of us are not there yet. By that, I mean we haven't lost our driver's licenses, our homes, the use of our legs, or our memories. We don't have to take 20+ pills a day and live by someone else's schedule. Neither our meals nor our clothes are chosen for us. Can you imagine working your whole life just to have everything taken away? I thought about that question a lot on days I wanted to lose my temper, or when I was in the mood to fight because my reality was the right one, and theirs was just plain wrong.

Then one day I learned that some days the person you're caring for just needs to talk. They don't need to have a discussion; they don't need your opinion. They just want to be heard.

I've had the privilege of caregiving for several family members over the last decade: my late father, my grandfather, and my grandmother. When I started caring for a non-relative, for Mrs. Bennett, she was recovering from surgery, and her family needed someone with a flexible schedule. She used a wheelchair. A series of UTIs (urinary tract infections) had induced a temporary demented state. This position was six months long. In that time, Mrs. Bennett and I became, what I would call, good friends. And just when I thought I knew everything there was to know about caring for someone, I'll be damned if the Divine didn't step in and teach me a little bit more. Praise for the art of listening, for it is indeed a true art. And thankfully, it's a learned skill, too—one that I work hard to do more of these days.

I think most people had stopped paying attention to Mrs. Bennett altogether when I got onboard. This was because of the dementia the UTIs had induced. She talked nonstop. It was an active and exhausting task to listen to her.

I was only scheduled three hours a day, though, which made me "fresh," and ready for whatever the illness had in mind (for I knew I'd be leaving eventually). I'd get my break. I'd be free. But even knowing that my time with Mrs. B. was finite, didn't keep me from playing on my phone while nodding periodically, or escaping to the kitchen to grab a glass of water. I used that excuse frequently. You see reasoning with her was out. Interrupting to add my two cents to a story was impossible. Basically, I was down to two options: ducking out for water, or feigning interest while playing on my phone.

Nobody was in the house but the two of us during my daily visits. It probably wouldn't have mattered if I had hid the whole time; I guess that could have been option number three—hiding in the bathroom. Mrs. Bennett talked nonstop with or without someone present. And there was no one around to tell on me. It was just me and my (recovering) Catholic guilt. Ah…so there was someone, or something in the room. This irritating emotion took hold and eventually begged the question: *Are ducking and dodging or playing with your phone your only choices? Really?* The answer was no. I guess they weren't. I could always suck it up and listen to the lady. That was my other choice.

The next morning as I took a nice deep breath and got past the dread zone, I promised myself I'd suck it up and listen to Mrs. Bennett no matter what she had to say.

I planted myself on the couch with my ears on high alert. There would be no reading, texting, checking e-mail, or getting on Facebook. I was going to listen. I'd join in the conversation when invited, but knowing that to rarely be the case, I settled in to simply listen to her.

I've spent so much time in my history of caregiving talking loved one through dangerous situations, holding their hands, rubbing their arms, hugging them if necessary, or coaxing them back to a safe zone, that I forgot about the power of stillness, of simply being with another person. It was time, that day, to set my busy schedule aside and take note of the words coming from Mrs. Bennett's mouth. I wasn't going to ask her if she wanted a foot massage, or if her coffee needed refilling, or her pillow fluffed. I had decided to devote an hour a day to Mrs. B. Even though no one was "looking," I was going to be listening.

Mrs. Bennett loved watching TV. She had her shows. Sometimes, rarely, but sometimes she dosed off. Mostly she talked to the TV, not necessarily about the topic of the show, often about what was on her mind. It was the *Judge Judy* hour. Mrs. Bennett adored Judge Judy, like they were best friends from kindergarten—lifelong buddies.

"They think they know me. They don't know me," she chirped angrily to Judge Judy.

"They think I'm nuts. Who knows, maybe I am nuts. But they don't know."

She took a long sip from her coffee. Then she held the cup in her jittery hand. It was no longer hot, and less than half full, so I let it quiver. I didn't want to interrupt.

"Maybe they're nuts."

"I never would have left if I knew all this would happen. I would have stayed in my own house with my pink couch and my pink curtains. I love the color pink. It's my favorite color. If the heat's too much get out of the kitchen! Everybody knows that. Even a fool knows that."

Mrs. Bennett smiled like she had a secret.

"You know that, don't you, Judge. If the heat's too much get out of the damn kitchen. Ain't nothing pink in the place I'm in now. It's all beige. Beige ain't even a color."

I chuckled. She had a point.

"In the Bible it says, don't think to highly of yourself. Debra gave me this Bible; she's my friend. She wrote a special Psalm out to me because she's my friend and I miss her, and it says; don't think too highly of yourself. Debra knows, but they don't know."

She set her coffee back on her TV tray.

"They all think they're something else. Well, the Bible tells you you're not! Do you hear me?" She slammed one fist into the other.

I was glad she didn't slam it on the table. Her skin was thin; she bruised easily. Mrs. B. paused to catch her breath. Maybe she was silently counting to ten, cooling down. She cocked her head at the TV.

"It ain't none of your goddamn business, Judge Judy, how many kids that woman has. I think five it too many damn kids too, Judge, but it ain't none of your damn business."

I chuckled again. This time she acknowledged it. She shifted her body a bit in my direction. She didn't make eye contact; she just subtly changed her body language to acknowledge me.

"I love Judge Judy. She is a smart, smart lady. But I sure as hell wouldn't want to be in her courtroom. She'll bulldoze right over ya." Then she pointed a crooked finger at the screen. *"You get her, Judge!"*

I was thinking the same exact thing.

"People are stupid. They all think they know me. They don't know me. I worked all my life. Every day. Went to work and saved my money. I bought myself a diamond ring. You think I don't have trinkets. I saved and saved and bought myself a diamond. I don't need no goddamn man. You want a diamond? You go to work, and you get yourself a diamond. You don't need no man. Course, I don't have to tell you that, Judge. You're a workingwoman. I bet you got yourself a diamond that's bigger than mine."

Judge Judy cut to a commercial. Seemingly satisfied, Mrs. Bennett closed her eyes. The break was brief. As soon as Judge Judy's voice emanated from the TV, she was up.

"I loved my daddy," she confessed to Judge Judy. *"I had the nicest mom and dad anyone could ask for. That picture right*

there," she said, pointing to a 4X6 in a brassy frame sitting next to the TV. "That's on their fiftieth wedding anniversary. I didn't have a driver's license until I was fifty-five. I rode the bus to work and took care of Mom and Dad, and when they died, I got my license."

I did not know that.

"I don't know where Judge Judy lives," she said, turning to me, "but I bet she's got herself a real nice house, a real nice house to go with her diamond."

I nodded, and was tempted to Google Judge Judy's house, but didn't.

"What makes them so smart, Judge? They didn't work their whole damn lives. I did! I worked! I saved my money and I deserve more. I deserve some damn dignity. I deserve my pink couch, or maybe just some curtains to spruce up the place. I deserve fried potatoes and real cream in my coffee. This creamer is for the birds! It ain't even real! It didn't come from a cow, it came from a factory, or some damn box. NASA. Maybe they make it in their labs! It's a science experiment gone wrong, that's what this shit is. What happened to real creamer?"

She gave her coffee a tiny shove. Then looked back at it, snatched it up, and gulped down the rest.

"And I don't think too highly of myself. I'm smart. I'm not nuts. I'm smart, and I like my trinkets, and they can all kiss my ass. And the color beige can go to hell. You hear me, chair? Go to hell!"

Mrs. Bennett was mad, but she caught her breath again, and with it, control of her temper. I could tell her humor was winning out, like I had often seen it do.

"If I lived by you, Judge, we'd be friends. We'd be best friends. You're sensible. I wouldn't want to get caught up in that courtroom of yours, though. No way."

Then she chuckled and trailed off…until she finally dozed off in her beige recliner.

I had no idea Mrs. Bennett owned a diamond ring that she purchased for herself. How empowering, I thought. I didn't even know a woman could do that— buy herself a diamond ring. She, too, was a caregiver…. Wow, I didn't know that. She didn't drive until she was in her fifties. That must have been scary and taken a lot of courage. I never knew she had a best friend named Debra, or that she even read the Bible. We never talked about religion. I don't know why.

It's amazing how knowledge is right there in front of us. I grew wiser that day. Wisdom wants to be found like a colored egg at Easter. It's all around us, in so many forms, just begging to be scooped up. But we have to calm ourselves on the inside and get out of our own heads to find it. Free our minds and our hearts to open the window for wisdom.

What I learned about Mrs. Bennett that day made me not only a better caregiver, but a better human being.

I learned to listen when no one's looking.

Five Caregiving TIPS from Jazz!

1. LISTEN to their stories. Everyone loves to tell stories, but it's no fun if you don't have someone who wants to listen.

2. PLAY GAMES…and even let them win! (…But only occasionally.)

3. PROMISE them ICE CREAM if they'll get undressed for the SHOWER. I'd get naked for ice cream! Just sayin'….

4. TREAT them NORMAL. I know it's not normal to wear two bras at the same time, well, that's what my mom said, but if you pretend it's normal, they don't feel so bad.

5. Say prayers with them at night. I love when Mom and I SAY our PRAYERS TOGETHER. It's more fun that way.

What Now?
Life After Caregiving

As I read Jazz a bedtime story, tears showered her book. They were streaming that freely from my puffy eyes—the eyes that I thought would be dry as dirt by now. It had been four days since Gram had died. It was her time. Her passing was a good thing, really. Still…. The grief had been attacking in waves every few hours since Nora Jo left this world, and it crept upon me fast and with a big undercurrent. Needless to say, the tears seemed to have a mind of their own, traveling in packs down my cheeks like armies of ants.

They (whoever "they" is—the experts) said I'd feel relief. When someone who is gravely ill dies, it's supposed to bring relief. That had not been my experience thus far.

When my father died from cancer—bald and seventy pounds under weight—*They* said he would look like his old self in my memories. *They* said that would happen real soon. Soon took one year. But it did happen, and that's how I see him now. So, I was waiting for the relief to set in. But after just four days, there was none. It must have been too soon.

I woke up this morning easy enough. But as I crept down the stairs to make Jazz breakfast, I turned and yelled in a whispery voice, "Be quiet when you come down, sweetheart! We don't want to wake G.G.!"

As soon as the words escaped my lips, it was as if the biggest bully on the playground had punched me in the gut. I grabbed my stomach with one hand, the wall with the other because I thought I was going to puke. When that feeling passed, I nice big jolt of "crazy" hit. And then after that, I waited and waited without moving an inch. I was waiting for the big blow, for Jazz to yell back, "Mom, you silly head! G.G.'s dead!"

There was nothing but silence, which meant Jazz must not have heard me. She's like my conscious; she'd never let something like that slide. I concluded she wasn't paying attention. Thank God.

Anyway, that's how I started day four of my new life without G.G. I was ending it by reading to Jazz with tears streaming ferociously down my cheeks, speckling her book, wrinkling its pages.

"Mama, Mama? Are you okay?" she asked.

"I'm okay, babe. I just miss G.G."

"Don't cry, Mama."

"It is okay, baby, it's okay to cry. It's okay to miss people." That was the best explanation I had. I mean, I had been crying for four days. I had forgotten the woman was dead twelve hours earlier. I was an f'ing mess.

Without saying a word, Jazz ran to the window, pulled back the curtain, looked up at the sky, studied it, and then leapt back into the bed.

Then she spewed out *this* speech:

"You know what I think; I think it's going to be okay, Mom. And I bet when we look up in the sky, the brightest star will be G.G. Tonight's not a good night, though, 'cause I can't see any stars; I just checked. But on a real starry night, me and you, we'll go outside and look up and she'll be there. And we can wave to her. She was eighty-nine. I wish she lived to be ninety-nine. But if I know G.G., she's gonna be the brightest star up there so we can always look at her. Does that make you not so sad?"

It made me not so sad.

I had asked God on several occasions that year—her final year of life—to please take my gram before Alzheimer's disease did the job. After all, she was declining. She hadn't said my name since last Christmas. She thought I was her sister most days, if she thought I was anyone at all. I also asked God if it would be all right (if it was cool with Him) if she could die in her home, *in our home,* amongst family. Nora Jo was a major homebody, nearly agoraphobic. I wanted her to be comfy till the end. And then I went so far as to ask Him to give me strength—an extra dose of it when that time came. I thought for sure I was screwed—going for the trifecta of wishes and all. But He granted every, single one.

When we first moved Gram in, people always asked the same question: "How long do you plan to keep her?"

I used to say a year. But after more than two years of caregiving, I had decided to revise the statement. "My plan is to take care of her...that's my plan," I'd say.

And we took care of her, not considering future options. Then one day when I wasn't looking, I'll be damned if God didn't grant all three wishes: She died of complications eight days after a heart attack. It was in our home because she would have never survived surgery, and the Alzheimer's ruled out the possibility of rehab. And even though I did spend three nights on a tile floor next to her bed, and zero nights sleeping, and hospice suspected me of taking her painkillers because I was that twisted up from grief, I survived it. I cared for her until the end. (Thanks again, God, for getting me through.)

They came fast, those wishes. She lived with us till death. She died of something other than Alzheimer's. She died in our family home. She didn't die peacefully in her sleep, though. (I clearly wasn't specific enough.) She spent the last week in excruciating pain with five compression fractures in her spine and two fractured ribs from a heart attack that did not kill her on the spot. Because she was honestly too weak for heart surgery, they released her to us. It seemed unimaginable to bring her home at the time. But because our doctor thought she had less than six months, hospice stepped in, and, quite frankly, saved us. They were angels—like Jazz—extinguishing the fear, exhaustion, insanity, and extra excess grief. As soon as any of that would spark, they'd snuff it out. If they weren't holding a hand, they were singing a song, changing sheets, or lending an ear. They wowed us all.

So, Nora Jo died not knowing me exactly, but she understood what my role in her life still was. And she died with her Jazzy by her side. It was difficult, but not impossible, because we did it.

If we can do it…. (Just sayin'….)

Hospice likened the "work of death" to the "labor of birth," and briefly, I understood the necessity of it all.

At the time, I thought I'd feel better when the winter clouds cleared, which would be in three months. When I could go outside with Jazzy, stand in the yard, and look for G.G.—the brightest star in the sky—that's when I'd be okay. Three months sounded doable.

I was right. Typically so, spring brought with it hope. That's when the road to recovery started. I'm still on that journey, however, over four years later. Occasionally, I'll smell Italian food, hear a joke, see a sign, and be reminded of Nora Jo. Three or four times since she's died, it felt like she came to me, like her soul trampled me down like a pack of phantom horses. I had to sit down. The missing her got the best of me; it came on that strong.

I will never stop loving that woman.

They should tell you that.

They should tell you that the pain will never leave, but that it will find a safe home inside your heart, and even make you stronger. The heartache will become your ally. It will make you believe in prayer, in living in the moment, and in the power of a Post-it note. It will remind you to hug a family member extra long the next time you say goodbye or to give a stranger a compliment 'cause it looks like they could use one. And even if you look crazy doing it, it will remind you to wave hello to the brightest star in the sky.

BONUS TIP #26

When all else fails, and all goes wrong, and you feel trapped in a fight that will never end, feel free to use our secret weapon: BETTY.

Betty is the make-believe woman we blamed for everything. Her name fell out of my mouth in an effort to calm Gram down from a squabble one day…and it stuck after that. If socks were lost, money was stolen…Betty did it. If hearing aids were missing, dresser change was gone, and the Nutter Butter bag was but a mass of crumbs: Betty. If it's raining, snowing, the tomatoes didn't ripen, the dogs won't stop barking, or the coffee tasted like mud…Betty. Betty was responsible for bad weather, barking dogs, and being an inadequate host. That bitch Betty, as Gram so fondly referred to her, was even the reason she had to shower….

Betty: Don't dig your way out of a fight without her.

Just the TIPS!

5 TIPS to Get Organized

1. Clutter clear
2. Familiarize them with the new surroundings
3. Create space just for them
4. Make a special spot in main living area
5. Give them their own counter space in kitchen

10 Safety TIPS

6. Signs
7. Baby gates
8. Safety locks
9. Keep dangerous things in high places
10. Keep useful items at eye-level
11. Segregate pets
12. Nightlights
13. Use plastic glassware
14. Hide alcohol
15. Hide prescription drugs (in high places)

10 TIPS for Surviving Caregiving

16. Laugh
17. Journal
18. Find "me" time
19. Plan a regular date night
20. Exercise
21. Have back-up available
22. Pray
23. Hold onto at least one hobby
24. Socialize (both of you if possible)
25. Vent when necessary
26. Betty

5 Caregiving TIPS from Jazz!

1. Listen to their stories
2. Play games with them
3. Have ice cream!
4. Treat them normal
5. Pray with them

Alzheimer's Association Facts and Figures

- Over 5.2 million Americans are living with Alzheimer's
- 36 million people worldwide have a dementia-related illness
- 15.5 million caregivers are unpaid totaling 17.7 billion dollars' worth of care (2013 Statistic)
- Over 60% over caregivers are women
- Over 67% of people with Alzheimer's are women
- Additional healthcare costs from the stress of caregiving totaled 9.3 billion dollars in 2013
- More than 19% of female Alzheimer's caregivers had to quit their job to care for a loved one
- Alzheimer's is the most expensive condition in the nation. It's estimated to cost the American society 214 billion dollars in 2014
- More than 33% of caregivers report depression. Its main cause is lack of sleep

Acknowledgments

My family and I cared for my grandmother, Nora Jo, for six years total…three years fulltime in our home—a million *thank yous* don't begin to express my gratitude to them.

As a former actor, I was totally unprepared for the trials of a dementia-related illness. For starters, as a former actor I was qualified for basically nothing that had to do with "care" or "giving." I wasn't ready for late nights, all nights, being stalked (in my own home), answering the same question 100 times a day, dealing with lots of tears, even more beers, and naked-ness. Gram forgot all about privacy and censorship. And my daughter was two when we moved her in. She learned a lot of new words, to say the least! And we lost some family because of our decision to have her live with us. But we gained things too: New friends. This illness drove away those that didn't quite get it and dragged in a crop of folks whose realities were far more flexible. These new friends dug her raunchy, repetitive style of storytelling. They loved to hear her sing, they held her hand when she cried. They didn't mind that she never knew who they were. They weren't embarrassed to be around us, at our home or in public. They adapted to our "Archie Bunker in really great drag." Thank you, Comrades in Compassion. You made her journey so special.

Finally, when we started getting good at caregiving, Gram passed away. But, she didn't pass before I was able to film her for almost two months. I filmed and interviewed her, and it was amazing. It became *14 DAYS with Alzheimer's.* Thank you, Ken Atchity, for your insight, direction, patience, mentorship, and friendship for the last fifteen years. Thank you. I never would have turned these homespun movie clips into a film without your keen eye and tutelage. With your assistance, I was able to create a tangible, lasting memory of my gram, and a film that has created a new kind of awareness for Alzheimer's disease and caregiving. On a personal note, I can pop in the movie and be one with her spirit for a whole 29 minutes when I get lonely. You made that possible, Ken. Thank you.

One thing worth mentioning: I regret not having more pictures. I have very few photos of Gram and me together. When I was deep in the madness of it all, I needed reminders like this from others, so I'm passing this one forward: Don't be worried about whether you've showered or if your makeup is in place. Take pictures, lots of pictures. You won't regret it. My friend, Barbara K. Pursley, put together the most beautiful photo collection—*To Mom with Love*—of her mother over her decade-long battle with Alzheimer's. Check that out on YouTube if you'd like photo journaling ideas: *Embracing the Moment: An Alzheimer's Memoir.* YouTube: http://www.youtube.com/watch?v=wJlEfr23Xec

Thank you, Danielle Canfield, for all your hard work on this project. Your energy, strong work ethic, attention to detail, and organizational skills turned these stories into a published book. You are my left-brain; I stand by that statement. And your kind, generous, and delightful spirit is why Jazz has already asked you to be her maid of honor—you know, someday....

Thank you to my mother, Sheri, who has always been my cheerleader. You read this and gave me great notes. Thank you, Mumsy. And, like a mother, you've always had an acute sense of what I need before I've even bothered to express it in words. I have a long list of packages (with stories to accompany them) that have mysteriously come through the mail over the years as evidence of your psychic mom abilities. Thank you for all you do.

And, Jazzlyn Jo Weaver....

Jazz,

You are my queen, and always will be. Thank you for choosing me as your mom. You are the youngest caregiver I've ever met—my born caregiver, my daughter, the love of my life: my darling, Jazz. I never could have done this without you. You're the reason I care, the reason I write. You're my reason. Thank you for being my favorite everything.

I love you,
Mom

About the Author(s)

LISA CERASOLI was a series regular on daytime's *General Hospital* when she got bit by the writing bug. In 2003, she left LA for Michigan to take care of her dying father. She stayed in Northern Michigan after his death to get married, become a mom, focus on her writing career, and care for her grandmother, Nora Jo. *On the Brink of Bliss and Insanity* was published in 2009 by Five Star Publications with the memoir *As Nora Jo Fades Away: Confessions of a Caregiver* following in 2010.

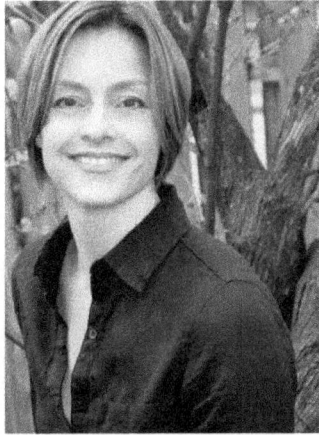

The books have garnered ten national and international awards. *Nora Jo* has a foreword by Leeza Gibbons, calling it Alzheimer's *Tuesdays with Morrie*. Lisa also directed and produced the documentary short *14 DAYS with Alzheimer's* with Ken Atchity executive producing. The film has received honors from 16 film festivals and has been shown in 50+ facilities all over the country where Lisa has spoken on the subject of caregiving. Lisa is the founder and president of 529 Books: A Full Editorial and Book Design Company (www.529books.com) and she's the VP at Story Merchant Books (www.storymerchant.com). She is a ghostwriter, screenwriter, writing coach, and assists writers at all levels of publishing.

JAZZLYN JO WEAVER, born June 1, 2005, was named after her grandpa, Jack Weaver, who used to play sax in a jazz band in Detroit. Her middle name is in honor of Nora Jo, of course. Jazz became a caregiver when she was just two and a half years old.

G.G. and Jazz were not just great-grandmother and great-granddaughter, but best friends, the biggest of rivals, and more like sisters in the end. Jazz taught G.G. how to play *Go Fish* when she could no longer remember the rules. They loved coloring contests even though Jazz despised losing, which was usually the case as G.G. was exceptionally good at staying in the lines. Jazz was the reason Gram got out of bed in the morning, and always the first person to dry her tears with a funny joke or silly dance. Jazz is the reason "Mommy" pulled this whole thing off.

Jazz is thirteen now. Her favorite sport is basketball. She trains daily and plays yearly with her school, tournament teams, and a traveling AAU team. She loves dogs. She's the proud parent of two Yorkie Poos, Feebie and Mocha. And, in her downtime, she's a sitcom junkie to the point that she's become Mom's producing consultant on the half-hour pilot for television she's developed with Ken Atchity based on the *Nora Jo* memoir.

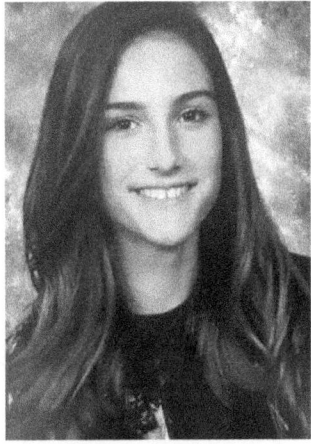

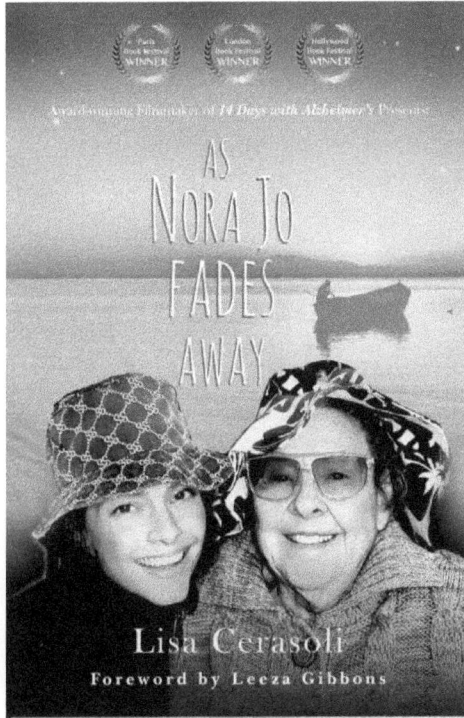

AS NORA JO FADES AWAY: Confessions of a Caregiver

Winner Paris Book Festival
Winner DIY Los Angeles Book Festival
Winner London Book Festival
Winner Hollywood Book Festival

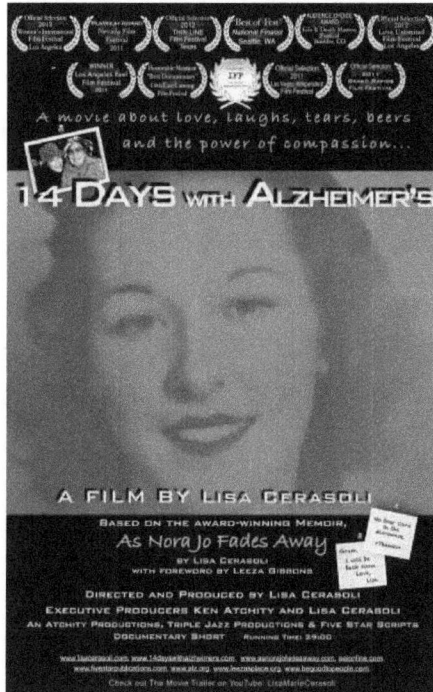

14 DAYS with Alzheimer's Awards:

Win: Best of Fest: Seattle National Film Festival Award 2013
Winner: Randy Becker TV Web Series Competition, 2013
Audience Choice Award: Life & Death Matters Festival, CO
Win: Los Angeles Reel Film Festival
Official Selection: Independent's Film Festival, Tampa, FL—
Chosen as A&E Documentary Selection
Official Selection: LA Women's International Film Festival
Official Selection: Las Vegas Independent Film Festival
Official Selection: Thin Line Festival, Texas
Platinum Award: Nevada Film Festival
Official Selection: Grand Rapids Film Festival

Official Selection: Detroit Windsor Film Festival
Official Selection: Life Fest Film Festival, Los Angeles
Official Selection: Green Bay International Film Festival
Official Selection: Love Unlimited Festival, Los Angeles

H.M. Best Documentary, 14th Annual East Lansing Film Festival
Incorporated by Columbia University into the Graduate Medical
Program: Topics in Nursing, Palliative Care

14 DAYS with Alzheimer's MOVIE TRAILERS can be viewed on
YouTube Channel: Lisa Marie Cerasoli

LINK to the full movie: *14 Days with Alzheimer's*, a 29-minute
Documentary: http://vimeo.com/28065118

For complimentary review copies of *As Nora Jo Fades Away*
write: lisacerasoli@gmail.com

14 DAYS... Movie Stills

A Story about Love, Laughs, Tears, Beers, and the Power of
Compassion.
A Film By:
Lisa Cerasoli
Executive Produced by Ken Atchity and Lisa Cerasoli

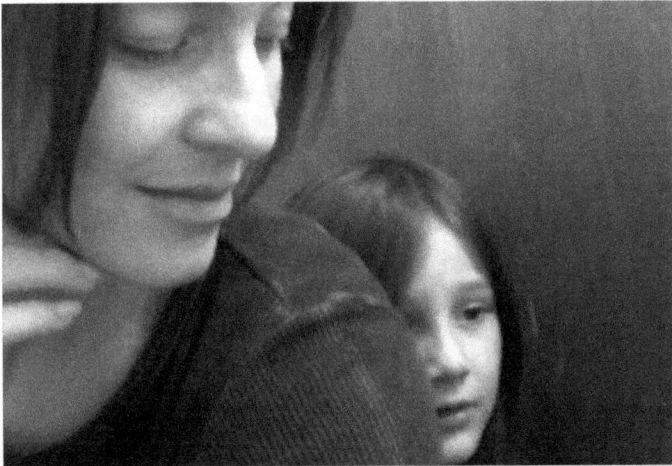

Lisa finds Jazz hiding in the bathroom. They talk about things they
loved about G.G., and then sing her favorite song: "Let's Make
Believe That We're Happy" by Kitty Wells.

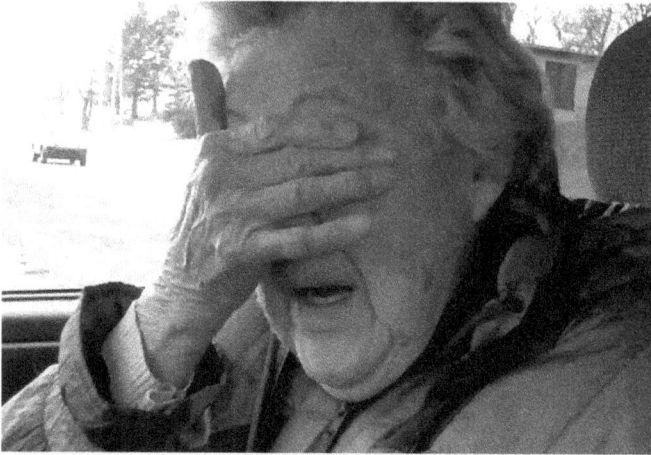

Nora Jo was told by an outside, part-time caregiver that Fritz, her husband of sixty-seven years, is dead after spending an hour looking for him. We "insiders" knew better than to tell her but were grocery shopping and came home to the situation. (We always told people to "go along" with her to avoid this kind of heartbreak, but you can't be everywhere all the time as a caregiver.)

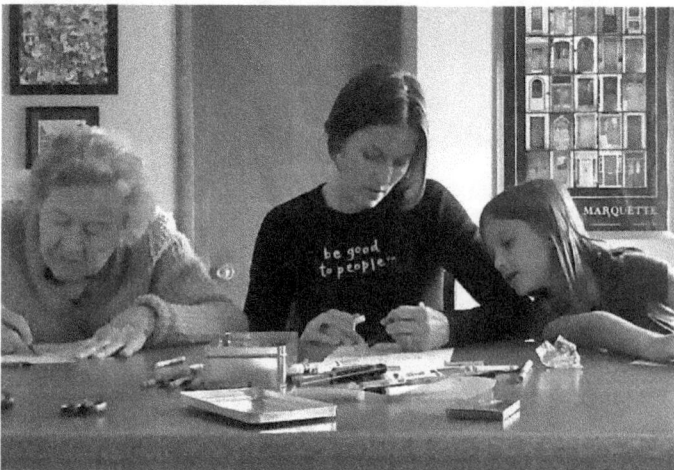

The Infamous Coloring Contest. G.G. took the gold ribbon that day.

25 TIPS

for

SURVIVING ALZHEIMER'S

Your Story HERE:

Your Story HERE:

Your Story HERE:

www.ingramcontent.com/pod-product-compliance
Lightning Source LLC
Chambersburg PA
CBHW032117280326
41933CB00009B/874